ATKINS DIET: 50 LOW CARB RECIPES FOR THE ATKINS DIET WEIGHT LOSS PLAN

JEFF ANDERSON

TABLE OF CONTENTS

Broccoli Chicken with Alfredo Sauce

Pork with Ginger and Coconut Milk

Simple Atkins Pancakes With Sausage and Bananas

Ricotta Goat Cheese with Walnuts

Atkins Potatoes with Chicken

Tasty Low Carb Fruit Kebabs with Almond Extract

Easy Atkins Recipe with Dijon Mustard

Low Carb Beef with Vegetables

Mozzarella Cheese and Sausage Pizza

Baked Chicken With Mushrooms and Oregano

Low Carb Beef Fajitas with Cilantro

Spaghetti with Parmesan and Greek Yogurt

Salmon with Oregano Flakes and Vegetables

Low Carb Beef with Oyster Sauce and Fresh Ginger

Simple Low Fat Salad

Beef with Cheese and Worcestershire

Atkins Boneless Chicken Breasts with Dried Parsley and Lime Juice

Low Carb Atkins Chicken With Mushrooms

Tasty Pudding Desert - Cottage Cheese

Atkins Pancakes with Meat of Your Choice

Meat Balls with Plum Sauce

Atkins Mustard Chicken with Yogurt

Spinach Fettuccini Shirataki with Beef

Vegetarian Shirataki Noodle Soup

Low Carb Eggs with Basil Leaves

Spanish Delight with Chili

Simple and Tasty Green Smoothie with Broccoli

Atkins Baked Pork with dills

Atkins Salmon Burger with Fat Free Fromage

Tasty Blueberry Kale Smoothie

Oat Bran Balls with Goji Berries

Dessert – Vanilla Cookies

Dessert - Chocolate Oat Bran Muffins

Atkins Bread with Fat Free Yogurt

Super Chili Bowl

Broccoli Salad

Easy Crackslaw

Bacon Wrapped Avocados

Parmesan Crusted Chicken with Bacon

WHAT IS THE ATKINS DIET?

The Atkins Diet is one of the most popular diets of all time with millions of people around the world claiming that it has made a difference in their life. It focuses on increasing the amount of protein that you consume, along with reducing your carb intake. The primary focus of the diet has to do with being hypersensitive to carbohydrates that are problematic. By reducing carbohydrates, our weight should also reduce, or, at least, that is the theory.

The Atkins Diet is now seeing resurgence as many experts are looking at this diet in a new way. If done correctly, this diet plan can be a healthy life style change. Yes, a healthy life, plus a new way to look at food. You can view the Atkins Diet as your way to shed those extra pounds you cannot seem to shake off no matter what exercise or diet you have tried. Sometimes, it seems like no matter what you do, you just cannot achieve the ideal body that you want. The Atkins Diet is your solution.

For those of you that are looking to lose more than just five or ten pounds, the Atkins Diet will allow you to lose a large amount of weight in just the first two to three weeks, with no strenuous exercise necessary. Your body itself will be doing all the work for you. The rest is learning how to keep the weight off and continue to eat healthy. This, in turn, will help you keep those extra pounds off for life.

We can look at the Atkins Diet as a new beginning in properly eating to become healthier. When you research and learn more about the Atkins Diet, it is safe and actually gives you the results you want. We first need to come to the conclusion that our enemy is the carbohydrates and not the fats. If we eat the right carbs in the right amounts, we can lose weight and keep it off for good.

Why Carbs Are Bad for You

Carbohydrates are the main source of energy for our bodies. Athletes need carbs to perform well and keep their energy up, meaning that the Atkins diet is seemingly impossible for those type of people. For the average person, the problem occurs when the carbs you are intaking come from a sugary, fatty coffee early in the morning. A small amount of the carbohydrates are used for energy, while the remainder is stored as fat deposits for later use.

Our bodies have this primeval programming that someday, we might be left in a desert and will need to store energy in the form of fat for future use. Sadly, the body over compensates and stores more fat than we need. We are consuming far more sugar than our body is able to process and that is the main problem. When the body is presented with fats and sugars, it takes the body more energy to burn fats we consume than to use the available sugars that we have consumed prior.

The Atkins Diet Today

Nowadays, many health experts from around the world are calling departments of health to change their advice, amending the carbohydrate myth, and telling people to eat a low-carbohydrate diet instead of a low-fat one. Most diets tend to fail because you are constantly being told to curb your calories, thus reducing the bulk of food you eat, causing you to feel hungry all the time. **With the Atkins Diet, you are only reducing the carbohydrate intake, not your total food intake.** With the Atkins Diet, **you are not counting calories.** You are, rather, counting the number of carbohydrates you can eat. Therefore, you can eat more and not feel hungry.

Sugar not only causes weight gain, but it is also highly addictive. Sugar causes a number of dangerous diseases that damage the body and impact how the brain functions. With our brain being made of 60% fat and with the ever persistent trend of cutting back on fats, it is no surprise that the elderly seem to be suffering from more degenerative brain diseases now more than ever. Later, we will discuss why this may be shown to be true in the future. It is also no wonder we are seeing more and more cases of brain disorders.

The following introduction to the Atkins Diet will guide you through each of the four phases, showing you how to lose weight effectively.

Staying Committed to the Atkins Diet

Your commitment will be rewarded.

Once you make the decision to follow the Atkins Diet, you will need will power and discipline to maintain it. The reason the diet has been so successful is because it does not require you to make sacrifices as big as other diets.

All you have to do is reduce certain types of foods in your diet. The 'induction' stage is only the first phase of four phases if you follow through with the whole diet. Consuming the exact amount of carbohydrates required per day is not easy, however referring to the recipes in this book will help.

The idea is to be consistent and then you will start seeing results within a short while. One way to stay motivated is to think of the end result. Every time you visualize an outcome, you are more likely to stay on course.

The 'Induction' Phase

In the Atkins Diet, the body will first start depleting the stores of energy located mostly in your muscles and liver called Glycogen. Glycogen is a carbohydrate that your body produces to have readily available in the event that you do not consume any carbohydrates and you need an energy source immediately.

When we restrict the consumption of carbohydrates, especially simple sugars, the body has to go and start using the emergency stores of Glycogen. After the body uses up all the stored Glycogen, it goes to your lipid cells or fat cells for energy.

When the body burns this form of energy source, it produces a byproduct called Ketones. These Ketones can be measured in the urine using a product that can be purchased at any pharmacy called Ketostix. There are different brands out there and it even comes in a generic form. Ask your local pharmacist and they will guide you in the right direction. Measuring the Ketones in the urine is how you know the fat burning process has begun. This is the jump start we had mentioned earlier. The burning of fat and production of these Ketones is your jump start. This is something that you may become obsessed with at first, waiting for this to happen, but it is a good indication that you are doing the diet correctly. The best time of the day to measure is early in the morning when you wake up. The body will have been burning fat overnight and an accumulation of

Ketones will have occurred, causing a higher reading. It can be measured during the day, but a weaker reading may be seen since you may have been diluting it from the fluids that you have consumed during the entire day.

Do not stop there. Follow through with the whole diet plan as it will teach you how to keep unwanted weight off. If you stop there, you may risk having the pounds return. People have complained of gaining their weight back, but that is because they did not follow through with the whole diet plan. See the plan through and stick to it.

Unlike other diets where we are restricting the calorie count, here, we are restricting the amount of carbohydrates. In the calorie-limiting diet, people often stop the diet because they are constantly hungry. With the Atkins Diet, you are not restricting the calorie intake or the amount of food you can eat, but rather you are restricting the carbohydrate amount. This way, you are able to eat more of the foods that keep you fuller longer because it takes the body longer to digest proteins and fats.

You may experience some sugar crashes where you may feel down and tired, but this will quickly change as the body begins to burn your own fat for energy. Once this process begins, it will deliver a steady supply of energy to the body, so that you will not experience this feeling of a lack of energy or motivation. Unfortunately, you may experience that crash initially, but think of it as your sugar detox diet period. After this period, you will begin to see the steady flow of energy that the body will produce once it starts burning its own body fat.

Most of the weight is lost in this initial induction phase, so the up most strictness and commitment is required if we are to make the pounds disappear easier than you ever thought they would. The induction phase requires the most dedication because as we mentioned earlier, the combination of fats and sugar-rich carbohydrates is what got us to the overweight problem we have today. This phase generally takes about two weeks or until you are about 10 to 15 pounds away from your desired target weight. If done correctly, you will begin to experience a relatively fast loss of weight that should motivate you to continue.

At the end of this book, I will provide you with resources to low-carb recipes. You will be very surprised to see what these low-carb recipes look like. They will not seem like recipes for a low-carb diet at all. This diet has been tested and done by so many people that there is almost an endless number of low-carb recipes out there. So again, please be patient and strong-willed during these first two to three weeks because this is where you will see the biggest results in losing weight. In this phase, you will see the biggest transformation on your body. This is generally why some people tend to stop here because they have already lost the weight and are happy with their results. If you do not adopt this diet as a lifestyle, the weight will come back because you will eventually go back to your old ways of eating. The rest is learning how to eat right for life. Once you accept this diet plan as a healthy way of eating, learn what to eat and what to stay away from, the rest is just keeping the pounds off.

TIPS ON THE 'INDUCTION' PHASE

Planning is key

Another critical aspect of this diet is to plan ahead. You will need to go shopping for the ingredients necessary to prepare or put together your two-week menu. Buy these groceries separate from what the rest of your family will be consuming. Notice that as these two weeks proceed, you will start to see the weight come off gradually, and this will begin to encourage you more and more to continue towards your goal. Try to have tunnel vision while in this phase. Be strong and avoid temptation. The satisfaction at the end will be incredible.

Don't Skimp on Fats and Protein

Eating sufficient proteins in every meal is paramount. It is important to keep the body from breaking down your muscles for energy. Instead, you need your body to use consistently your own body's fat for a steady source of energy. Try to include about 4 to 6 ounces of proteins or fats per serving each day. There are no carbohydrates in meats, so that may be a good choice.

Remember that protein does not only come from meats. Proteins can come from other sources too, like beans. Lentils are also very high in protein. Learn to keep these foods in your diet if you are not familiar with them. Experiment with other sources of proteins, like cheese, to keep your diet interesting.

With the Atkins Diet, certain foods have no limit and will keep you fuller longer. These foods also provide a more steady flow of energy versus the rise and crash of simple sugars. Bear in mind that most of these carbohydrates should come from the foundation veggies. As for dairy, you can eat 3 to 4 ounces of cheese per day. Substitute your milk for almond or soy varieties for now, but it will be introduced at a later phase. *When substituting milk, do not forget to read the label for added sweeteners.*

Sugar is Your Enemy

Fruits and grains (like bread and pasta) are not allowed during the induction phase. Although fresh fruit and nuts are very healthy food to consume, they are not permitted during the induction phase because they are high in carbohydrates and simple sugar. Remember, in this stage, we are restricting sugar as much as possible. Be patient. Fruits will come in the later stages. The Induction phase is just two weeks, and you will be moving on before you know it. Starchy vegetables, like potatoes, are also a taboo. Right now, we are focusing on controlling the carbohydrates, so that we may lose the weight and then, reintroduce certain foods back in a healthier way.

Be on the lookout constantly for hidden carbohydrates, especially in prepackaged food. Be very vigilant. The food industry will mask sugar in all kinds of names, predominantly as corn syrup. Take the total carbohydrates listed on the label and subtract the fiber content, and that will give you the net carb.

It is encouraged to have three meals and two snacks each day during this phase of the diet. Keeping your meals balanced between 18 and 22 grams of net carbohydrates can be tricky at first, but try to stay within this range as best as possible. Do not deviate too much from the range given. A variation of about 3 to 4 grams up or down would not make a big difference, but do not splurge one day and try to compensate for it on another day. This will only slow down the process. Stay with the course in these crucial first two weeks. Be strict and precise.

Hydration and Supplementation

Stay hydrated by drinking about 8 eight ounces of water daily or more, if possible. During the induction phase, you will lose some body weight in the form of water, which is normal. Water is also critical to prevent constipation, especially in this stage. Sodium intake is also important at this point because while you are losing water, you may also be losing sodium, which could be a cause for the lack of energy and possibly, the lowering of blood pressure. Some of this fluid can come from things like coffee, tea, or other acceptable beverages. A good source of sodium is the use of soy sauce as part of the flavoring for some of your meals or consuming regular broth, not the low sodium brand.

Add vitamins and mineral supplement to replace any vitamins or minerals that may be flushed out in the initial days when you are losing water weight. When choosing a supplement, make sure to read the label and avoid brands that put sugar in their product to make it more palatable.

THE 'ONGOING WEIGHT LOSS' PHASE

The primary goal of the 'ongoing weight loss' phase is to find your own critical carbohydrate level for losing weight. The critical carbohydrate level is the amount of carbohydrates that you will be consuming until you find the total number of carbohydrates that do not cause weight loss or weight gain. We will do this by experimenting with different foods from the step approach to food that is going to be discussed later. The various steps will guide you on how to know which foods and in what quantities you can consume to keep the weight off.

How To Find Carb Sweet Spot for You

In the 'ongoing weight loss' phase, we will continue to do everything we were doing in phase one, but we will be gradually adding about 5 grams of carbs with other higher carb foods while continuing to lose weight, but at a slower rate. We may see ourselves adding grams of carbs and consuming as high as 35 to 45 grams of carbs and still be losing weight. We started with the limit of about 20 grams per day, but now, we will gradually add 5 grams of different foods as stated above. As we move up on these steps, the carb content will continue to increase, so it must be done gradually to see how the body reacts. There is no limit to how high your carb intake should be.

Just as the 'induction' phase was necessary to lose the initial weight, this stage is very important because it will teach you how to eat in order to keep the pounds off. This phase is where many people will quit instead of learning how to eat properly, so they can continue this pattern for the rest of their lives. Stick with it and learn it.

There is no straight answer as to how many carbohydrates to consume because everyone is different. There are many factors that vary from person to person, making it hard to determine a universal carbohydrate consumption number. The important thing to keep in mind is to do it 5 grams at a time. In the 'induction' phase, we lose weight fast. Our goal here is to lose weight slowly until we are within 5 to 1o pounds of our target weight. At this stage, we will be gradually approaching our desired weight and learning what is our own individual balance of carbohydrates that we can consume, and in what quantities, so we do not gain or lose weight. By the end of this phase, and especially the next, you should be a pro at learning what foods your body want. In other words, you will know which foods to consume and which to stay away from.

In this phase, we will be gradually adding nuts, berries, and some starchy vegetables. We will still keep the foundation of carbohydrates at 12 to 15 grams daily and we will still need the eight ounces of water or acceptable drinks per day. The more water we drink, the better. Keeping the body hydrated is very important. We will be continuing the 'induction' phase, but we be adding carbohydrates with a step-ladder approach. **The step-ladder approach means that we will be adding carbohydrates**

slowly according to the different steps on a scale. The higher we go on the scale, the higher the carb count. Start with the first group and move up onto the scale and see how your body reacts to each group as you progress. Remember that in this phase, we want to continue to lose weight, but at a much slower pace. We will be testing each of these food groups to see how we react to them.

THE 'TUNING' PHASE

The goal in the 'Tuning' phase is to reach our target weight or be about 5 pounds from it. The 'Tuning' Phase may be the simplest phase in the whole Atkins Diet. We can view it as a continuation of phase two, but here, we have already spent lots of time in phase two, testing how our body will react to the different foods in the step ladder of food groups.

In the 'Tuning' Phase, we will be experimenting mostly with foods on the last two or three steps of the food group pyramid. These are the ones with the highest carbohydrate count, so we really need to be careful with the amounts of these foods we consume. We do not want to suffer a huge set back. Let us increase it again about 5 grams at a time and decrease by 10 if the weight begins to come back. If we are consuming any prepackaged foods, do not forget to read the label. To find the net carb, subtract the total carb from the fiber content. Net carbohydrates are what we are always counting when looking at any prepackaged food. Anything you pick up, read the label. By now, we should have gotten the hang of it and should know how to increase or decrease the amount of food we consume to continue losing weight.

THE 'LIFETIME MAINTENANCE' PHASE

You are in the 'Lifetime Maintenance' phase, which simply means you have already made it to your target weight and have been there for about a month. The Atkins Diet, if followed as instructed, is a healthy, lifelong diet. You will have times when you may gain a few pounds, but now, you have the know-how on what to do to keep them off. Remember, carbs are what got us in trouble, so always be vigilant of your carbohydrate count and keep it in check.

The body will instinctually go back to releasing insulin and storing those carbs into fat. A combination of fruits and vegetables, in the appropriate amount, mixed with the appropriate amount of healthy fats and protein will make for a lifelong diet that you can always follow. If you choose to go the route of processed foods, which I do not recommend, but can be done, always remember to read the label. There are many ways in which the industry hides the word 'sugar,' mostly in the form of corn syrup.

WHY THE ATKINS DIET IS A GREAT CHOICE

The Atkins Diet is a perfect diet for fast-paced and busy lifestyles. You will lose weight without any exercise. Your body will be doing all the work for you. If you do not follow the Atkins Diet word for word, you will not lose weight. There is no calorie counting, or strict exercise regiments. Committing to the Atkins Diet does not take time out of your daily routine; rather, it is a slight alteration in your way of eating. All that is asked of you is to stick to the diet plan as strictly as possible. Eventually, the types of foods that you can eat and in what quantities will become second nature; you will automatically know what to do.

Although I probably would not recommend exercising during the 'induction' phase because the amount of carbohydrates that the body is using for energy is being restricted, I would, on the other hand, recommend waiting for one of the ladder phases. That way, you will be more familiar with the diet plan and therefore, can focus and introduce an exercise plan that will fit your schedule. The Atkins Diet has to do with knowing what you can and cannot eat, in accordance with your carbohydrate count. You need to become a carb detective in everything you consume by reading every label.

Reduce Blood Pressure, Prevent Diabetes

We are all very tired of hearing and are very aware that obese individuals have a higher risk of heart disease, cancer, high blood pressure, breathing problems, Type II diabetes, and other conditions. For those with Type II diabetes, the Atkins Diet is a great way to keep the diabetes under control. When you eat carbs, your body breaks them down into sugars. In Type II diabetes, there is too much sugar for the body's insulin to break down, which leads to some serious medical problems. If less carbs are consumed, there is less sugar in the blood, resulting in the diabetes being under control. Imagine that - no more finger pricking to read blood sugar levels. No more having to inject yourself with insulin because your sugar levels are low. On the Atkins Diet, your body will not require the insulin anymore.

Even better, you will not have to deal with, or at least prolong, the long term effects of living with high levels of sugar in the blood. Some of these long term problems include, loss of eye sight or in more extreme cases, losing a finger or two. The long term high sugar levels in the blood stream will cause the body to lose sensation to the hands, fingers, and toes. With the Atkins Diet, you will be eating a healthy diet and keeping the sugar levels down and hence, reducing the possibility of having such complications.

Other studies related to the Atkins Diet have shown a direct correlation between weight loss and a decrease in blood pressure for hypertensive patients. **Weight loss means lower blood pressure and a reduced risk of heart disease and atherosclerosis. Overall, you will experience better heart health.**

This healthy diet is not just about changing the way you look, but rather, a weight loss plan to help you live a longer and healthier life. That is why it is worth the commitment. We can go on and on about the benefits of this diet on our health, but we should not be looking at just the immediate results of the diet, but the long term effects on our health.

Proof of Commitment

There are no cheat days on the Atkins Diet. If you break the diet and binge on carbohydrates, you can add up to 5 pounds in one day. Although some of this is from water retention, it may take up to a week to get back on track with your weight loss. Some people get nauseous and feel horrible when their carb level increases after staying away from carbs for so long. Sometimes, breaking the diet leads to super strong carb cravings, which can make it even tougher to follow the diet. **If you cheat one day, do not give up.** You can get right back on track, however, it is easier to just say "no" to those mashed potatoes at Thanksgiving dinner. Be strong-willed. **People will respect you more when they see the new and healthier you.**

Psychological Approach to Weight Loss

Just because you are on a diet, does not mean you have to be miserable! You will need to make small adjustments to the way you approach your meals. If you are a pasta lover, find low-carb vegetable pastas. As mentioned earlier, I will provide you with some resources to low-carb recipes that may seem familiar to you already, but will be altered in the carb content. The whole idea is to make a two week plan for what you will be eating during the 'induction' phase. This way, there is no guessing. You know exactly what your meal strategy will be. Put this plan in writing. Draw up a diagram or list of what you will be eating for breakfast, snacks, lunch, and dinner. Today, there are thousands of recipes on the internet that you can create and that are very simple. You do not need to be a chef, in order to create delicious low-carb meals. Many recipes are just putting some ingredients together.

Speaking of ingredients, **as soon as you have a plan in writing, go to the super market and buy the specific ingredients you will need.** Stay strong and committed. Do not allow other family members to tempt you into buying processed foods that will set you back on your diet plan. Cheating will only deter you from weight loss. When your family sees how you have slimmed down in such a short amount of time, they will want to do the same. In no time, the whole family will want to follow your eating habits. **An alternative to cooking all your meals is to buy them already made. There are frozen Atkins meals that are now sold almost everywhere.** The trick is to plan ahead. Stick to purchasing only the ingredients that you will need for your weekly diet plan. This will ensure success. It is simple.

THE END OF OUR JOURNEY IS YOUR NEW BEGINNING

We have made it to the end. Your journey to your transformation is now complete. You finally have the tools necessary to succeed in creating the new you. Remember, whether for health or to lose those stubborn pounds, by reading this far, it tells me you are committed to this diet. The only thing left is to execute the diet plan. Make it your mission of a lifetime to accomplish this hurdle. You and your loved ones will be very proud of you.

You must be committed and know that the Atkins Diet is a healthy diet if done correctly. There is no room for cheating here and there. Any deviation from the correct course will only delay the ultimate goal. At first, it may be a little difficult to follow, but you will get there.

The word 'diet' sometimes has negative connotations, so that is why we will eventually no longer look at it as a diet, but a way of life. Stay strong during the 'induction' phase. It is where you will lose the bulk of your weight and after that, it is mostly about keeping the weight off. Imagine if you were one of those people that have been trying to lose weight for years and cannot seem to find the way how. The Atkins Diet has been around for many years now and has been tried and tested with surprising results. The Atkins Diet will help you lose those pesky pounds, will encourage you to want to keep them off, and get you feel good both physically and emotionally. I guarantee that you will lose weight during the 'induction' phase without any physical effort, except for the effort you put into sticking with the diet plan.

You will be able to do activities that you may have shied away from in the past. You may meet new people, surprise your doctor, and maybe have the motivation to get involved in some exercise program that can further help your weight loss. I clearly saw it in my wife and myself. When she saw those pounds coming off, she seemed as if she was determined to lose more weight than me and tone her body. She was now looking for that muscle to shine through. The feeling is intoxicating. Just make the effort to get started and you will be gaining the intent to lose weigh and look and feel excellent.

Remember to read labels. Sugar is masked in many names, predominantly as corn syrup. **Beware of low fat.** Most products that say low fat are not necessarily healthier for you because they are usually loaded with sugar or salt to enhance the flavor of the food.

Cheese and Baby Spinach Quiche

Ingredients:

- 2 Tbsp. butter
- 10 eggs
- 1 c. heavy cream
- 8 oz. shredded cheddar cheese, sharp
- 1/2 tsp. black pepper
- 10 pieces bacon
- 2 c. baby spinach, fresh
- 1 c. onion, chopped

Directions:

1. Bring out the slow cooker and grease the bottom with some butter. Turn it on to the low setting and let the remaining butter sit on the bottom. This will allow it to melt while you work on getting the rest of the ingredients ready.
2. Next, you will need to cook the bacon. The method used for this is not too important as long as you are able to save the bacon grease to use when you are done.
3. Take the spinach and cut the stems from it before chopping into pieces that are about half an inch long. As you are tearing, place into a measuring cup to get the amount that is needed. Chop up the onion as well.
4. Bringing out a bowl, beat the eggs inside before whisking in the onion, spinach, pepper, cheese, and cream. Make sure that these are all well combined. Pour this mixture inside the slow cooker when done.

5   Tear up the bacon into small pieces, about half an inch for the pieces, and then top the mixture in the slow cooker with the bacon.

6   Place the cover on the slow cooker and let the mixture cook for about 5 hours on a low setting or 2.5 hours if on a high setting. When the quiche is firm to the touch, it is ready to eat right away.

Atkins Low Carb Egg Breakfast Pie

Ingredients:

- Diced yellow onion
- 1 Tbsp. garlic powder
- Pepper
- 8 whisked eggs
- 1 shredded sweet potato
- 1 lb. pork sausage
- Salt
- Tsp. dried basil
- Peppers of choice

Directions:

1 Take out the slow cooker and grease it with a little bit of coconut oil in order to ensure the eggs do not stick to the slow cooker.

2 Next, take the sweet potato and shred it up. You can use a shredder or place the sweet potato into the food processor and shred it that way.

3 Take the sweet potato into the slow cooker along with the rest of the ingredients and then mix them together well with a spoon.

4 Cover the slow cooker with the lid and place it on a low setting for about 8 hours. Make sure that the eggs and the pork sausage are cooked all the way through. When the dish is all done, slice it up like a pie and serve warm.

Low Carb Apple Oatmeal

Ingredients:

- 2sliced and peeled apples
- 1 tsp. cinnamon
- 1/3 c. brown sugar
- 2 c. rolled oats, old fashioned
- 4 c. water
- Pinch of salt

Directions:

1   To start this recipe, take out the slow cooker and use a liner, the brown sugar can make a big mess and this can help with clean up.

2   Take the apples and slice them up before placing along the bottom of the slow cooker. Sprinkle the cinnamon and the brown sugar on top of the apples, and then use a spoon to stir it all together until well mixed.

3   Take the oats and pour them all over the apples before adding some salt and water over it all. It is not a good idea to stir it all together since it is going to mix together when it cooks.

4   Place the cover back on the slow cooker and then place it on a low setting for about 9 hours. You will be able to let this cook overnight so that it is ready when you wake up. If you are not ready to eat breakfast when you get up, just turn off the heat and let it stay warm until you are ready.

5   When you are ready to eat, stir it all together well in order to get the oats unstuck from the bottom. Serve warm and enjoy!

Atkins chicken garlic Chowder

Ingredients:

- 2 diced celery ribs
- 6 oz. sliced cremini mushrooms
- Sliced sweet onion
- 4 garlic cloves
- Chopped shallot
- Sliced leek
- 1 c. heavy cream
- 1 lb. bacon tsp. salt
- 1 tsp. pepper
- 1 tsp. garlic powder
- 4 Tbsp. butter
- 2 c. chicken stock
- 1 lb. chicken breasts, boneless and skinless
- 8 oz. cream cheese
- 1 tsp. thyme

Directions:

1 Begin this recipe by bringing out the slow cooker and turning it on to the low setting. Add in the pepper, salt, 1 cup of chicken stock, 2 tablespoons of butter, onions, mushrooms, celery, leek, shallot, and garlic inside. Cover the slow cooker and let the vegetables cook for an hour.

2 While the vegetables are being cooked, bring out a skillet and pan sear the chicken in the rest of the butter.

You will want to cook for around 5 minutes on each side or until the chicken is browned.

3   Take the chicken out of the pan and set it aside. Use the rest of the chicken stock to de-glaze the pan and scrap off any of the remaining bits of chicken that have gotten stuck to the pan. Cut up the chicken and then add the chicken stock and the chicken to the slow cooker.

4   At this time you can add in the thyme, garlic powder, cream cheese and heavy cream to the slow cooker. Stir all ingredients together well so that there will no longer e any chunks of the cream cheese present. Add the bacon into the slow cooker lastly.

5   Add the cover back on to the slow cooker to cover and then let it all cook for about 8 hours or until done. Serve warm.

Tasty Chipati Wraps

Ingredients:

- 1 lbs. turkey cutlets, chopped up
- 1 tsp. minced garlic
- 1 tsp. cumin
- 1/2 tsp. cayenne pepper
- 1/2 tsp. coriander
- 1/2 tsp. ground ginger
- 1/8 tsp. cinnamon
- Dash cloves
- 8 chipatis

Directions:

1 To begin this recipe, bring out a bowl and combine together the cloves, cinnamon, ginger, cayenne pepper, cumin, garlic, and turkey strips. Allow this mixture to stand in the side for a few minutes while you are working on the other ingredients.

2 Next, bring out a grill pan that will fit on your stove and spray it with some vegetable spray before heating up for a few minutes on a medium high heat. Place the turkey strips onto this grill and allow them to cook for about 5 minutes or until the strips have time to be lightly browned and they are done. When the strips of turkey are done you can take them from the grill and remove to a clean bowl.

3 Place the chipatis or paleo approved tortillas onto the grill, just placing two at a time. Let them set on the grill

for around 3o seconds on each side before transferrin over to the cutting board.

4   Open up the tortillas and place the turkey inside. You can add some of your favorite paleo approved ingredients for toppings into the tortilla. Fold this in half and then enjoy.

Green Beans with Jalapeno

Ingredients:

- 1 tsp. lemon juice
- Salt
- 2 Tbsp. canola oil
- 1 bag frozen green beans
- 1 onion
- 1 Tbsp. cumin seed
- 1 jalapeno

Directions:

1   To begin this recipe, bring out a pan and place the cumin and the oil inside. Allow the cumin to roast for about 3 minutes on some medium heat or until down. At this time you can add the onion to the pan and let it continue to sauté for a few more minutes until it is golden brown.

2   Add the pepper, salt, and frozen beans in at this time. Taste the dish before turning the heat up to high, put the lid back on, and allow it to cook for another to minutes. You can add in the lemon juice after this time if you would like.

3   Take the time to cook until this becomes the right consistency that you would like.

Afghan Peas with Chicken and Turmeric

Ingredients:

- 200 g. chicken breast
- 1 c. chopped onion
- 1 c. chopped tomatoes
- 3 garlic doves
- 3 spoons tomato paste
- 1 c. canned green peas
- 1 c. water
- Salt
- Curry
- Garam masala
- Turmeric

Directions:

1   To get started on this dish, bring out a pan and place the onion and the oil inside. Allow the onion to fry until it has time to turn a light gold color. At this time you can add in the garlic and then the chopped thicken. Keep on mixing until the chicken as time to become lightly cooked.

2   Place the tomatoes in with this mixture and let it cook for a few minute minutes while you are mixing. Add in the peas and the tomato paste along with a little bit of water to keep it all working. Add in a little bit of salt of

the taste that you like. Garam masala and turmeric are also nice additions.

3   Cover the pan and allow the whole dish to continue cooking until it becomes tender. Serve this right away.

4   At this time you can add in the thawed spinach and let everything come back to a boil. Toss the chopped herbs, raisins, and lime juice in for the last thing.

5   When you are ready to serve you can serve with the yogurt and decorate with some of the mint leaves that you had set to the side.

Low Carb Chicken and curry

Ingredients:

- 6 chicken thighs, boneless and skinless
- 2/3 c. miracle whip light
- 1 can cream of chicken soup, healthy request
- 1 tsp. curry powder

Directions:

1   To begin this recipe, take the Chicken and rinse it off before patting it dry. Bring out your slow cooker and get it all set up the way that it needs to work. When the slow cooker is ready you can place the chicken inside, trying to keep it all in one single layer the best that you can.

2   Next, you can bring out a bowl and mix together the rest of the ingredients. When they are well combined you can pour this mixture all over the chicken as evenly as you can.

3   Place the lid on the slow cooker and allow the dish to cook on a high setting for around 5 hours. Stir it gently right before serving and enjoying.

BROCCOLI CHICKEN WITH ALFREDO SAUCE

Ingredients:

- Jar three cheese
- Alfredo sauce
- 1/2 lbs. chicken breasts, boneless and skinless
- 8 oz. whipping cream
- Broccoli

Directions:

1   To begin this recipe, bring out a slow cooker and place the chicken at the bottom. Bring out a bowl and mix the whipping cream and the alfredo sauce together. Pour this mixture on top of the chicken.

2   Place the lid on top of the slow cooker and let it all cook together for about 41/2 hours on a high setting. You will know the meal is done when the chicken is cooked.

3   Pull the chicken out of the slow cooker. Shred it up before returning the slow cooker and letting it stay warm. Steam the broccoli before serving it with the chicken mixture and enjoying.

PORK WITH GINGER AND COCONUT MILK

Ingredients:

- 2 tsp. salt
- Tbsp. olive oil
- 3 Tbsp. minced lemon grass
- 2 lb. pork
- 2 inch ginger
- 2 garlic cloves
- 1 Tbsp. apple cider vinegar
- 1 tsp. pepper onion
- 1/2 c. coconut milk

Directions:

1. Take the extra fat from the roast, making sure to leave a little bit. Slice a crisscross pattern onto the top layer of the pork.
2. Mince up the garlic and then slice and peel the ginger up. Peel and slice the onion as well. Bring out a slow cooker and place the onion rounds into the bottom.
3. In a bowl, combine together the pepper, apple cider vinegar, minced lemongrass, garlic, salt, and olive oil. Mix until it starts to form a loose paste.
4. Rub this mixture on to the pork and then place inside the slow cooker. Cover and let it marinate overnight.
5. When you are ready to cook, place the slow cooker inside the pot and then add in the coconut milk. Let the mixture cook on a low setting for about 8 hours.

6   After this time, shred up the pork with a few forks and then serve warm on a bun or with your favorite side.

Simple Atkins Pancakes With Sausage and Bananas

Ingredients:

- Large egg
- 1/12 cup pumpkin
- 1/24 cup cottage cheese
- 1/12 tsp. pumpkin spice
- 1/24 cup of almond flour
- 2/3 oz. protein powder
- 2/3 Tbsp. soy flour
- 1/6 tsp. baking powder
- 1/2 small banana
- 2 Tbsp. almonds
- Turkey sausage

Directions:

1   Mix the protein powder, flower, baking powder, eggs, cottage cheese, pumpkin, canned pumpkin, and almond together until both the egg and the pumpkin are well blended.
2   After all of this is mixed together, preheat a skillet on medium heat and drop in the batter on the heat, making the pancakes as large or small as you like them.
3   Once the bubbles start to form on the batter it is time to flip the batter over and cook for another 2 minutes.
4   While the batter is cooking, cook up the sausage in another skillet. When everything is cooked, place the

pancakes and the sausage on a plate along with the sliced banana on top.

RICOTTA GOAT CHEESE WITH WALNUTS

Ingredients:

- 3 Tbsp. Parmesan eggs
- 12 spinach leaves
- Cooking spray
- 1 cup ricotta cheese
- Goat cheese
- 3 Tbsp. walnuts
- 2 Tbsp. basil
- Salt
- Pepper

Directions:

1 Heat up the oven to 350 degrees and use the cooking spray to coat the custard cups. While the oven is heating up, combine the pepper, salt, egg, basil, walnuts, parmesan, goat cheese, and ricotta together and mix.

2 Line the custard cups with a couple of spinach leave and divide up the cheese mixture. Bake the cups for about 3o minutes and then cool for 5 minutes.

ATKINS POTATOES WITH CHICKEN

Ingredients:

- 14 1/2 oz. chicken broth
- 1/2 cup white wine
- Instant potatoes
- 1 tsp. Thick-It-Up

Directions:

1. Combine the Thick-It-Up and the broth together in a bowl. After you are done with that you can heat up the wine on high heat and cook until it has been reduced by about 1/3, which will take about 1 minute.

2. Once that has been done you can combine the broth mixture into the wine and bring it all to a boil until it thickens, which will take another 2 minutes. Serve together with your favorite meal.

Tasty Low Carb Fruit Kebabs with Almond Extract

Ingredients:

- 2 kiwis
- 1/2 cup blackberries
- 8 strawberries
- 16 raspberries
- 1 star fruit
- 1/4 cup cream
- 3/4 cup yogurt
- 1/2 tsp. almond extract
- 1 1/2 Tbsp. sugar substitute

Directions:

1 Take a skewer and put on 1 star fruit slice, 2 strawberries, 2 blackberries, 2 raspberries, and 1 kiwi slice on each one Once all of the skewers are lined up you can mix together the almond extract, sugar substitute, cream, and yogurt together before placing into a serving dish. Dip your skewers into the yogurt mix and then serve.

EASY ATKINS RECIPE WITH DIJON MUSTARD

Ingredients:

- 24 cocktail franks
- Tbsp. butter
- 6 Cuisine bread from Atkins
- 1/4 cup Dijon mustard

Directions:

1. Start by preparing the bread by trimming off the crusts and then brushing the bread with the butter on both sides and then cutting into four strips.
2. Take one of the cocktail franks and roll it up into each slice of break and poke it with a toothpick.
3. Heat up the oven to 350 degrees and arrange the side on the baking sheet before cooking for to minutes. Serve the appetizer hot and with some of the Dijon mustard.

Low Carb Beef with Vegetables

Ingredients:

- 2 cups celery
- 2 cups of water
- Garlic cloves
- 1 cup cabbage
- Tbsp. olive oil
- Stew beef
- 1 onion
- Tbsp. beef base
- 1 tomato, diced
- 1/2 cup carrots, chopped

Directions:

1   Heat up some oil in a skillet and then cook the onion and garlic together until they are tender and then set the mix aside.
2   Add some more of the oil to the skillet before adding the beef and browning it. Drain out the grease with the beef before adding the beef base and the celery, cloves, cabbage, carrots, and tomato.
3   Cook the mixture on the low setting for an hour to an hour and a half.

Mozzarella Cheese and Sausage Pizza

Ingredients:

- Tbsp. olive oil
- 1 cup mozzarella cheese
- 1/2 of a red pepper
- 1 cups baking mix, all purpose
- 1 1/2 tsp. baking powder
- 1 packet sugar substitute
- 11/8 cup water
- 1/2 cup tomato sauce sausage link
- 1/2 green pepper
- Red onion

Directions:

1   Heat up the oven to 425 degrees and then blend the sugar substitute, salt, baking powder, and baking mix together in a bowl before adding the oil and the water.
2   Combine all of these ingredients into a dough and then place on a surface that is clean.
3   Use a rolling pin to roll out the dough to fit onto your pizza pan and then bake this crust for about 10 minutes. Remove from the oven and then spread out the tomato sauce, sprinkle on the mozzarella along with the onions, red pepper, green pepper, and sausage links.
4   Place all of this back in the oven for another 10 to 13 minutes, cut into slices and serve.

Baked Chicken With Mushrooms and Oregano

Ingredients:

- 1 1/4 chicken thighs
- Tbsp. olive oil
- 1/4 cup Baking mix, all purpose
- Salt
- Pepper
- 1/2 lb. mushrooms
- 1/4 tsp. pepper flakes
- 1 1/2 Tbsp. garlic
- 1 tsp. rosemary
- 1/2 onion, chopped
- 1/2 cup white wine
- 9 oz. artichoke hearts
- 1 1/2 tsp. oregano

Directions:

1   Start by preheating the oven to 350 degrees before placing the salt, pepper, and baking mix into a plate and mixing together. Take the chicken into this mixture and coat both sides evenly.

2   Heat up a skillet and then cook up the chicken for about 4 minutes or until it has browned a little. Add the onion to the chicken and sauté it for another 2 minutes before adding the mushrooms and sautéing for another 3 minutes.

3   Next add the garlic and stir in for around 3o seconds before stirring in the red pepper flakes, rosemary, artichokes, and wine and then bring to a simmer. Pour out this mixture onto the chicken that has been placed to the side and then bake it all for about 4o minutes. Season with oregano, pepper, and salt if you desire.

Low Carb Beef Fajitas with Cilantro

Ingredients:

- Cumin, grounded
- 1 Tbsp. canola oil green pepper red pepper
- Tbsp. olive oil red onion
- Garlic doves
- Tbsp. lime juice jalapeno pepper
- Steak
- 12 tortillas
- 3/4 c. sour cream
- 3/4 c. green salsa
- 1/4 cup cilantro

Directions:

1. Start by preparing the marinade; you can do this by combining together the olive Ingredients: oil, cumin, jalapeno, lime juice, salt, and garlic together in a large bowl.
2. Once that is done you can marinade the steak by letting it sit in the juices for no less than an hour. Heat up the oven to 350 degrees and warm up the tortillas for about 15 minutes.
3. After the hour has passed, take the steak out of the marinade and grill for about 3 to 4 minutes on each side. Next you will need to heat up the canola oil on a skillet in order to cook the onion and both bell peppers for about 5 minutes.

4   After the steak has been grilled you need to slice into thin pieces. Take the tortillas out of the oven and spread on the vegetables, cilantro, sour cream, steak, and salsa over them. Fold the tortilla over and then enjoy.

Spaghetti with Parmesan and Greek Yogurt

Ingredients:

- 1/4 tsp. lemon zest
- 1/2 tsp. lemon juice
- 1/4 c. Greek yogurt, non fat
- 1 1/2 Tbsp. Parmesan cheese, grated Salt pepper
- Salt
- Pepper
- Garlic cloves
- Shallot Cooking spray
- C. Cauliflower florets
- 1Tbsp. olive oil
- 1/4 tsp. garlic powder
- Prosciutto pieces
- Tbsp. olive oil
- Pinch red pepper flakes
- 9 Zucchini
- 1 Tbsp. minced parsley Lemon Dressing

Directions:

1   To begin this recipe, you can turn on the oven and let it heat up to 450 degrees. While the oven is heating up, take out a baking tray and line it with some parchment paper before setting aside.

2   Bring out a bowl and toss the cauliflower with some pepper, salt, garlic powder, and olive oil together. Lay

this cauliflower out on the prepared baking tray and then place into the oven. Let it roast for about 20 minutes or until it becomes pierced with a fork and is lightly browned.

3   While the cauliflower is cooking, bring out another bowl and combine together all the ingredients for your lemon dressing. Set this aside for a bit. Mince things and the garlic together before setting aside as well.

4   Bring out a skillet and coat it with some cooking spray before allowing it to heat up. Lay out the prosciutto slices on it. Let it cook for about 5 or until they become crispy. Transfer these slices onto a plate lined with paper towels and set aside.

5   Give the skillet time to cook down for a few minutes before adding in some olive oil. Let the oil heat up and then add in the red pepper flakes, shallots, and garlic. Cook for another 30 seconds so it becomes fragrant and then add in the zucchini noodles.

6   Cook this mixture for about 5 minutes, making sure that you toss frequently. When the noodles are al dente, add in the crumbled prosciutto and the cauliflower. Give it another toss and then take it from the heat. Stir the Greek yogurt mixture in and then give it another toss in other to combine completely.

7   Divide this mixture into some bowls, garnish with the parsley and serve warm.

Salmon with Oregano Flakes and Vegetables

Ingredients:

- 1 pinch oregano flakes, dried
- 4 oz. skinless salmon filet
- Drizzle olive oil
- 1 Tbsp. lemon juice, freshly squeezed
- 1 pinch red pepper flakes
- Garlic clove
- 1 Tbsp. vegetable broth
- 1 lemon wedge
- Salt
- Pepper
- 1 leek stalk
- Olive oil

Directions:

1. To start this recipe, turn on the oven and let it heat up to 425 degrees. While the oven is heating up, take out a baking sheet and line it with some parchment paper. Lay the salmon in the middle of the baking sheet and then drizzle on some of the olive oil. Splash a little bit of the lemon juice on top and season with the pepper, salt, and oregano.
2. Place the baking sheet into the oven and let the salmon bake for about 25 minutes. You will know

that the dish is done when the salmon flakes when you use a fork.

3. While the salmon is baking, bring out a spiralizer and cut up the parsnip before setting aside. Slice the leek thinly before setting aside. Mince the garlic as well and then set it aside as well.

4. About ten minutes before the salmon finishes up, bring out a skillet and turn it on to medium heat. Add in a little bit of olive oil and let it heat up. Once the oil is warm, add in the red pepper flakes, leeks, and the garlic. Let these cook or about 2 minutes so that the leeks can soften.

5. Add the parsnip pasta and the vegetable broth to the skillet. Cover the skillet and let it cook for about 5 minutes so that the parsnips have time to cook through.

6. Once the salmon is cooked through, bring out a fork and let it flake into small pieces. Add it to the skillet with the parsnip noodles, giving the skillet a good toss before transferring it to your serving plate. Serve with some lemon wedges and then serve.

Low Carb Beef with Oyster Sauce and Fresh Ginger

Ingredients:

- 1 oz. beef fillet
    - Onion, chopped
    - Tbsp. vegetable oil
    - Carrot chopped
- 1 green bell pepper (coarsely chopped)
- 1 tsp. fresh ginger root
- 1 clove garlic (minced)
- 1 Tbsp. oyster sauce
- 1 Tbsp. soy sauce
- 1 Tbsp. white sugar
- 1 Tbsp. of almond flour
- 1 Cup of beef stock
- Salt and pepper (to taste)

Directions:

1. Sauté beef over medium heat in a large skillet until browned, or for around 5 minutes,
2. Add garlic, onion, and ginger and sauté for another 5 minutes then add beef broth, carrot, and green bell pepper. Let mixture simmer after reducing heat to low. Combine cornstarch, flour, and oyster sauce in a bowl until the mixture becomes pasty. Add mixture to beef and vegetables and simmer until thick. Stir constantly.

3   Season with salt and pepper and proceed to serving.

Simple Low Fat Salad

Ingredients:

- Tbsp. of large capers
- Small red onion
- Bacon slices
- Medium tomatoes
- Ripe Avocado
- 10 cups salad greens
- Vinaigrette
- Croutons

Directions:

1   In a pan, cook bacon until crispy and drain on paper towels. Set aside. Make sure to leave fat in the pan. Once the pan is hot, add capers and saute for around 2 to 3 minutes. Take out the capers from the pan and drain on paper towels, as well.

2   Next, submerge the onion slice in a bowl of water and pat dry. In a large bowl, combine bacon, onion, avocado, croutons, and tomato with the salad greens. Sprinkle vinaigrette all over the salad and toss until well coated. Divide salad onto plates and top each with extra avocado slices. Serve and enjoy!

BEEF WITH CHEESE AND WORCESTERSHIRE

Ingredients:

- 1/2 cup water
- 1 cup of tomatoes
- Tsp. Worcestershire sauce
- Medium red bell peppers
- 1/3 cup of onion
- 500 grams of lean ground beef
- 1/2 cup long grain rice, uncooked dash salt
- 1/2 cup of cheese
- Pepper

Directions:

1. Remove membrane and seeds from the peppers and cut the tops off. In salted, boiling water, cook the peppers for around 5 minutes and drain on paper towels.
2. Add Parmesan cheese and a dash of salt inside the peppers.
3. Then, cook beef with the onions until beef turns brown.
4. Then, sprinkle salt and pepper all over the beef. Add water, tomatoes, Worcestershire sauce, and uncooked rice and simmer for around 15 minutes or until rice is tender.

5   Add cheese and stir. Stuff the peppers with the mixture that you have made and bake for around 25 minutes at 350 F. Serve warm and enjoy!

ATKINS BONELESS CHICKEN BREASTS WITH DRIED PARSLEY AND LIME JUICE

Ingredients:

- 3/4 teaspoon salt
- 1/4 teaspoon dried parsley
- 1/4 teaspoon thyme
- 1/2 teaspoon garlic powder
- 1/4 teaspoon onion powder
- 1/8 teaspoon cayenne
- 1/4 teaspoon black pepper
- Boneless chicken breasts, 6 pieces
- Tbsp. Lime juice
- Olive oil
- 2tsp Butter

Directions:

1. Mix the spices together.
2. Coat chicken with the spice mixture.
3. Place the butter and oil in the skillet over medium heat.
4. Sauté the chicken breasts until they are golden brown in color.
5. Using the remaining garlic powder and lime juice to season the chicken pieces.
6. Coat evenly while sautéing.

Low Carb Atkins Chicken With Mushrooms

Ingredients:

- Chicken, 1 cup of sliced lean meat
- Mixed mushrooms, 12 ounce
- Cream, 1 cup
- 1 teaspoon Garlic,
- Clove
- Bacon, 2 slices
- Chicken stock, 1/2 cup
- Brandy, 2 ounce Black pepper

Directions:

1. Heat oil in a wok over medium heat.
2. Add bacon and garlic then stir-fry until bacon turns golden brown.
3. Add the chicken and continue stir-frying until chicken becomes tender.
4. Set aside the chicken in a separate container and keep warm. 5. Using the same wok, fry mushrooms and spring onions until tender.
5. Add the chicken back in and continue to stir-fry for 5 more minutes.
6. Add the brandy, stock, and cream then bring to a boil.

7   Lower heat and allow the dish to simmer until the sauce decreases by half.

8   Season with black pepper.

TASTY PUDDING DESERT - COTTAGE CHEESE

Ingredients:

- Eggs
- 350 g low fat cottage cheese
- 1 teaspoon vanilla essence
- 2 tablespoons lemon juice
- Sugar substitute
- Cinnamon powder to garnish

Directions:

1. To the beaten eggs, add cottage cheese, vanilla and sugar substitute. Mix well.
2. Transfer to a lightly greased baking dish and bake for 45 to 50 minutes in a oven preheated at 160 degree C or until cooked to light golden brown.
3. Remove from oven. Cool before slicing and serve.

ATKINS PANCAKES WITH MEAT OF YOUR CHOICE

Ingredients:

- Oat bran
- 100 g virtually fat free quark
- Fat free fromage
- Eggs, separated, beaten
- Herbs of your choice
- Salt to taste
- Pepper powder to taste
- For filling flaked tuna/smoked salmon/ extra lean ham
- Cooking spray

Directions:

1. Mix together in a bowl, oat bran, fromage, quark, herbs, salt, and pepper. Add the egg white with the filling.
2. Spray a nonstick pan with cooking spray. Pour the batter.
3. Cook until the bottom side is golden brown. Flip sides and cook the other side too.

Meat Balls with Plum Sauce

Ingredients:

- 1/4 cup Chinese plum sauce
- Worcestershire sauce
- 1/4 cup rosemary, finely chopped
- Large onion, chopped
- Cloves garlic, crushed
- Eggs lightly beaten
- 1/2 kg beef, minced
- Basil, finely chopped
- Salt to taste
- Pepper powder to taste

Directions:

1 Mix all the ingredients. Shape into small lemon sized balls.
2 Place a nonstick pan over medium heat. Add the balls in batches and cook until they are golden brown.
3 Remove and place on paper towels for a few minutes before serving.

ATKINS MUSTARD CHICKEN WITH YOGURT

Ingredients:

- Chicken breast, skinless
- 1 ounce Dijon mustard
- 1/2 teaspoon thyme
- 1/2 teaspoon vegetable oil
- 1 ounce non fat yoghurt
- Salt to taste
- Pepper to taste

Directions:

1   Mix together in a bowl, chicken, mustard and thyme. Coat well. Let it marinate for io-15 minutes.
2   Line a baking tray with foil. Place the chicken on the tray.
3   Cover the chicken with another foil.
4   Bake in a preheated oven 300 degree C for 45-50 minutes or rill the chicken cooks.
5   Meanwhile mix together in a boil, yogurt, salt, pepper, and oil.
6   Remove the chicken from the oven and pour the yogurt mixture over it. Serve hot.

Spinach Fettuccini Shirataki with Beef

Ingredients:

- Packet Spinach Fettuccini Shirataki, cooked as per instructions on the package
- 1/2 pound grass fed ground beef
- 1/4 cup parsley, chopped
- Pepper

Directions:

1. Place a nonstick pan over medium heat. Add beef and pepper.
2. Sauté for 7-8 minutes until browned. Add noodles and parsley and cook for 4-5 minutes. S
3. Serve hot and enjoy!!!

Vegetarian Shirataki Noodle Soup

Ingredients:

- 750 ml vegetable stock
- 35g firm tofu, cubed
- 11/2 teaspoon ginger, minced
- Cloves garlic, sliced
- 150 g Shirataki noodles
- Scallions or spring onions, roughly sliced
- Spring onions or scallions, finely sliced for garnish
- Teaspoons soy sauce

Directions:

1 Pour vegetable stock in a saucepan. Place over medium heat.
2 Add tofu, ginger, and garlic. Bring to a boil. Lower heat and simmer for 5-6 minutes.
3 Add spring onions and soy sauce. Simmer until the noodles are cooked.
4 Serve in bowls and garnish with finely sliced scallions.

Low Carb Eggs with Basil Leaves

Ingredients:

- Eggs
- Small onion, chopped
- Cooking spray
- 200 g tomatoes, chopped (canned or fresh)
- Warm water
- Basil leaves, chopped

Directions:

1. 1.Place a nonstick frying pan over medium heat. Spray with cooking spray.
2. 2. Add onions and sauté until soft. Add tomatoes and water. Mix well.
3. Lower heat. Cover and simmer until the tomatoes thicken slightly.
4. Add basil. Mix well.
5. Now break the eggs on top of the tomatoes. Sprinkle salt and pepper. Cover again.
6. Cook until the whites are firm and yolk is still moist. Serve immediately.

SPANISH DELIGHT WITH CHILI

Ingredients:

- Packets frozen seafood
- 1 teaspoon extra virgin olive oil
- Cloves garlic, finely chopped
- Tomato puree
- Red chili, finely chopped
- Chives

Directions:

1 Place a pan nonstick pan over medium heat. Add oil. Add garlic, sauté until brown.
2 Add the seafood mixture. As the moisture evaporates, add salt and pepper. Sauté for a couple of minutes and add tomato puree.
3 Simmer for 5-6 minutes. Add chives and serve immediately.

Simple and Tasty Green Smoothie with Broccoli

Ingredients:

- 1 stalk celery
- 2 tablespoons chia seeds
- 2 cups cold water
- 2 packets dried wheat grass
- 2 tablespoon flax seed oil
- 1 cup frozen broccoli
- 2 cups Fresh or spinach
- 2 cups Kale
- 2 scoops Vanilla protein powder (optional)

Directions:

1. Blend all the ingredients until smooth. Serve with crushed ice.

ATKINS BAKED PORK WITH DILLS

Ingredients:

- 2 tablespoons dill
- 2 cloves garlic
- 500 g lean pork, cut into cubes
- 2 tablespoons parsley
- 1/2 green bell pepper
- 1/2 red bell pepper
- 1 tomato, chopped
- 1 medium yellow onion

Directions:

1. Mix all the ingredients together.
2. Place a foil over a baking sheet. Place the mixture over the sheet.
3. Cover with another foil to make into a pouch. Place in a pan of water. Place the pan in an oven.
4. Bake in a preheated oven at 180 degree C for 2 hours.

Atkins Salmon Burger with Fat Free Fromage

Ingredients:

- 4 tablespoons oats
- 2 eggs
- 1/4 cup fat free fromage
- 2 teaspoons baking powder
- 2 teaspoons mustard
- 2 ounce virtually fat free quark
- 2-3 tablespoons dill, finely chopped
- 2 slices smoked salmon

Directions:

1. Mix together in a bowl, oat bran, eggs, fromage, and baking powder to form dough.
2. Pour the dough in 2 round molds and microwave for 4 minutes,
3. Remove the buns from the mold and slice into 2 horizontally.
4. Spread mustard over one of the slice of each bun. Spread quark over the mustard.
5. Sprinkle dill. Place salmon on top. Cover with the other slice of the bun and serve.

Tasty Blueberry Kale Smoothie

Ingredients:

- 2 tablespoons almond butter
- 2 cups frozen blueberries
- Few cubes ice
- 2 cups kale
- 1 cup non fat vanilla yogurt

Directions:

1. Blend together all the ingredients until smooth. Serve in tall glass.

OAT BRAN BALLS WITH GOJI BERRIES

Ingredients:

- 4 tablespoons oat bran
- 1/4 cup unsweetened soy milk or fat free milk
- 1/4 teaspoon chia seeds
- 1/4 teaspoon flax seeds
- 10 goji berries
- Stevia to taste
- 2 tablespoons unsweetened coconut flakes

Directions:

1. Mix together all the ingredients in a bowl.
2. Shape into small balls. Roll in coconut flakes and serve

DESSERT – VANILLA COOKIES

Ingredients:

- 4 eggs, separated
- 1 teaspoon liquid sweetener
- 2 teaspoon vanilla extract
- 4 tablespoons oat bran

Directions:

1. Mix together yolks, vanilla, sweetener and the oat bran in a bowl.
2. Beat the egg whites rill they form stiff peaks.
3. Gently fold the whites into the oat bran mixture.
4. Pour on a cookie sheet. Bake in a preheated oven at 180 degree C for 15-20 minutes.

DESSERT - CHOCOLATE OAT BRAN MUFFINS

Ingredients:

- 12 tablespoons oat bran
- 2 tablespoons reduced fat cocoa powder (without sugar)
- 4 eggs
- 3/4 cup zero fat yogurt
- 2 teaspoons baking powder
- Sweetener to taste

Directions:

1. Mix together oat bran, cocoa, and baking powder in a bowl.
2. Add yogurt, whisk. Add eggs, whisk until smooth. Add sweetener.
3. Place paper muffin cases in muffin tray. Pour the batter (half fill the muffin cases) into the muffin cases.
4. Bake in an oven preheated at 175 degree C for about is minutes or until done.

ATKINS BREAD WITH FAT FREE YOGURT

Ingredients:

- 8 tablespoons oat bran
- 1 teaspoon baking powder
- 4 tablespoons fat free yogurt
- 8 tablespoons fat free cream cheese
- 4 eggs
- 1 teaspoon onion powder
- 2 teaspoons dried chopped onions
- 1 teaspoon garlic salt
- 1/2 teaspoon pepper powder
- 1 teaspoon Italian herbs seasoning

Directions:

1 Whisk all the ingredients together in a bowl until smooth.
2 Transfer the batter in a microwave dish and microwave on high setting for about 4 minutes
3 Remove it from the microwave and let it cool
4 Invert the dish onto a cutting board.
5 Cut into about 4 squares. 6. If you like it crunchy, then toast the squares in the toaster.

SUPER CHILI BOWL

Ingredients:

- 1 tbsp. Extra Virgin Olive Oil
- 2 peppers Jalapeno Peppers
- 1 tsp. Garlic
- 1/2 tsp. Salt
- 1/8 tsp. Cinnamon
- 1/4 tsp. Red or Cayenne Pepper
- 2 tbsps. Chili Powder
- 1 1/2 tsps. Cumin
- 2 lbs. Ground Beef (80% Lean / 20% Fat)
- 1 14.5 oz. can Diced Tomatoes
- 1 1/2 cups shredded Monterey Jack Cheese
- 1 medium (2-1/2" dia) Onion

Directions:

1. Heat broiler. In a 9 or 10-inch ovenproof skillet, heat olive oil over medium-high heat for 1 minute.
2. Add onion; cook until golden, about 3 minutes, stirring occasionally. Add garlic and jalapeños; cook 30 seconds, stirring until fragrant.
3. Add salt, red pepper, chili powder, cumin, cinnamon and ground beef to skillet. Cook until browned, about 6 minutes, stirring occasionally. Drain excess liquid from pan.

4. Add tomatoes, and bring to a boil. Sprinkle cheese over top. Place 5 inches from heating element, and broil just until melted, about 5 minutes.

BROCCOLI SALAD

Ingredients:

- 6 cups broccoli
- ⅓ small onion, chopped
- 1 cup mayonnaise
- ½ cup almonds, chopped
- 2 tablespoons red vinegar
- 8 slices cooked bacon, chopped
- Salt and pepper to taste

Directions:

1. In a large bowl, combine broccoli, bacon, onion, and almonds.
2. In a separate bowl, mix mayonnaise, vinegar, salt and pepper, in a small bowl.
3. Pour dressing over broccoli mixture and stir until evenly coat.
4. Cover and refrigerate for at least one hour or until ready to serve.

Easy Crackslaw

Ingredients:

- 1 lb. (450g) ground beef
- 2 minced garlic cloves
- ¼ teaspoon artificial sweetener
- ½ teaspoon minced fresh ginger or ¼ teaspoon ginger powder
- 2 tablespoons toasted sesame oil
- 1 teaspoon white vinegar
- 3 sliced green onions
- 14 oz. (400g) coleslaw mix (or shredded white cabbage)
- 2 tablespoons soy sauce
- ½ teaspoon hot sauce
- Salt and black pepper, to taste

Directions:

1. Brown the ground beef in a skillet and season it with salt and pepper to taste.
2. Remove the beef from the pan and set aside.
3. Drain off the fat if you wish.
4. Heat up the sesame oil and sauté the garlic, onions and coleslaw mix or cabbage in there until the cabbage is cooked to the desired tenderness.
5. Stir in the hot sauce, soy sauce, sugar or sweetener, vinegar and ginger.
6. Add the ground beef back in and mix well to combine.

7. Serve with hot sauce on the table for people who like it extra spicy.

BACON WRAPPED AVOCADOS

Ingredients:

- 4-6 Strips of Bacon
- 1 Avocado
- 1/3 Cup Brown Sugar
- 1/2-1 Teaspoon Chili Powder

Directions:

1. Heat the oven to 425
2. In a small bowl, mix together the brown sugar and chili powder. Set aside
3. Line a baking sheet with tin foil.
4. Cut open the avocado and remove the pit. Slice about 3/4" slices lengthwise through the avocado, and then cut through the middle to cut all of the slices in half so that you have thick chunks of avocado.
5. Cut each slice of bacon in 3-5 pieces and wrap each piece around the avocado. Roll in the brown sugar mixture and place on the baking sheet.
6. Bake at 425 for 10-15 minutes. Remove from the oven to a platter and stick a toothpick in each for serving.

PARMESAN CRUSTED CHICKEN WITH BACON

Ingredients:

- 1/2 tsp. salt
- 1-1 1/2 cups shredded Asiago cheese – for melting on top
- 3-4 slices bacon – cooked and crumbled (can leave slightly under-done, it will finish cooking under broiler)
- 1 egg beaten
- 1 tablespoon water
- Oil for frying – about 1/2 – 3/4 cup depending on size of skillet
- 4 boneless skinless chicken breasts – about 4-5 oz. each
- 1 cup grated Parmesan cheese
- 1/4 tsp. garlic powder
- 1/4 tsp. pepper

Directions:

1. Preheat oven to 350 degrees
2. In a small shallow bowl, mix egg and water
3. In another shallow bowl, mix Parmesan cheese, pepper, salt and garlic
4. Heat oil over high heat
5. Dip each chicken breast first in egg mixture then in cheese
6. Fry in hot oil until crust is golden brown
7. Prepare a baking pan by covering with foil and placing wire rack on top
8. Place chicken on rack and bake about 20 minutes or until juices run clear
9. Time will depend on thickness of chicken

10. Remove from oven and turn oven to broil
11. Top each piece of chicken with Asiago cheese and bacon and place under broiler to melt cheese

DESSERT - FROZEN CHOCOLATE WHIPS

Ingredients:

- 1 cup Heavy Whipping Cream
- 4 Tbsp. of Cocoa Powder (use 3 Tbsp. for a more milk chocolate flavor)
- 2½ Tbsp. Swerve Sweetener (these can also be made with sugar or other sweeteners, but you may need to adjust the amounts)
- ½ tsp. vanilla extract
- 1 pinch of sea salt

Directions:

1. Put all ingredients into a large mixing bowl and beat on high with the whip attachment until the whipped cream has firm peaks.
2. Transfer the chocolate whipped cream to a piping bag fitted with a 1M piping tip.
3. On a parchment lined baking sheet swirl the whipped cream around into large mounds like soft serve ice cream. Make around 12 or so and freeze on the baking sheet for at least 1 hour. They will be set at this point and you can eat them or transfer them to a freezer safe plastic tub for easy eating later.

ALMOND AND COCONUT MUFFIN IN A MINUTE

Ingredients:

- 1/8 cup Almond Meal Flour
- 1/3 tbsp. Organic High Fiber Coconut Flour
- 1 tsp. Sucralose Based Sweetener (Sugar Substitute)
- 1/2 tsp. Cinnamon
- 1/4 tsp. Baking Powder (Straight Phosphate, Double Acting)
- 1/8 tsp. Salt
- 1 large Egg (Whole)
- 1/3 tbsp. Extra Virgin Olive Oil

Directions:

1. Place all dry ingredients in a coffee mug. Stir to combine.
2. Add the egg and oil. Stir until thoroughly combined.
3. Microwave for 1 minute. Use a knife if necessary to help remove the muffin from the cup, slice, butter, eat.

ATKINS BROWNIES

Ingredients:

- 4 ozs Unsweetened Baking Chocolate Squares
- 1/2 cup Heavy Cream
- 5 large Eggs (Whole)
- 1 cup Sucralose Based Sweetener (Sugar Substitute)
- 1/2 cup Unsalted Butter Stick
- 2 tsps Baking Powder (Straight Phosphate, Double Acting)
- 4 1/2 servings All Purpose Low-Carb Baking Mix

Directions:

1. Pre-heat oven to 325°F.
2. Place the unsweetened chocolate and butter together in a bowl and microwave on high power for approximately 2 minutes until chocolate is melted. Whisk in heavy cream.
3. In a separate bowl, add the eggs and 1 cup of granular sugar substitute. Beat together using an electric mixer until mixture is just blended. Reduce mixer to low speed and then blend in the chocolate mixture.
4. With a wooden spoon, mix in the baking powder and 1 1/4 cups low-carb baking mix.
5. Coat 8 x 8 inch pan with non-stick vegetable oil spray and spread batter evenly into pan.

6. Bake at 325°F for 30-35 minutes or until done (toothpick inserted in the center comes out clean). (Do not over-bake or brownies will be dry and hard.)
7. Once cooled, cut into 5 rows by 5 rows to make 25 brownies.

FINAL NOTES

Thank you for downloading my book, Losing Weight without Dieting: Discover Weight Loss Secrets to Help You Lose Weight without Dieting! I hope you put everything you have learned to use and obtain the body you have always wanted.

If you enjoyed my book and wish to help me out, you can leave the book an honest review on Amazon.

You can also check out some of my other health and fitness books by visiting my author page on Amazon.

www.ingramcontent.com/pod-product-compliance
Lightning Source LLC
Chambersburg PA
CBHW062042280526
45788CB00003B/1073